MW00961234

High Protein Vegan Cookbook

Copyright © 2023 Evann Francis Ryan
All rights reserved.

The Meal Prep Plan

Welcome to month one of your high-protein vegan diet. I can't wait for you to reap the benefits of a well-balanced, satiating, and, importantly, a flavourful way of eating plant-based food. Going vegan has never been easier. There are plant-based alternatives at most grocers, and restaurants in most cities are getting on board with plant-forward menu options. There is still a long way to go in the education of not just switching to a plant-based diet but learning how to build a macronutrient-balanced plate for optimal health, digestion, and satisfaction.

Some benefits to eating a high protein diet include helping you naturally eat fewer calories, building more muscle mass, which can appear like better overall body composition, and the fact that protein burns more calories than carbs or fats simply digesting. Eating adequate high-quality protein boosts your hair, skin, and nail health!

The recipes focus on protein, but in the recipes, you will notice a good balance of carbs for energy and healthy fats for optimal health. Protein is great, but we need a good balance of protein and macronutrients.

At the beginning of each menu, you will see a macro breakdown for the three meals combined. Each recipe is meal prep for four days. The chosen

4-day meal prep keeps the meals fresh and exciting. If you do not want to cook every four days or you are meal prepping for two people, you can double each recipe to achieve eight meals.

The macros calculated are a rough estimate based on the ingredients used by the author and are not a personalized plan for your specific needs. Each meal showcases a balanced macronutrient breakdown of protein, carbs, and fats to assist you in making balanced meals. To note: The macronutrient breakdown calculated for the complete meal option is on each recipe page.

Each 4-day menu varies slightly in calories, carbs, fats, and protein. The calculated macronutrients will leave you room for some unplanned snacks or treats.

You will notice an *Increase the Portion* tip at the end of each recipe. This tip is available so you can customize this meal plan to fit you and your needs. For example, if you do not want to leave room for snacks or dessert, you can increase the portion of each meal.

In some recipes, you will notice an ingredient underlined -- a link to the specific brand used. When using a different brand, you will need to adjust the macronutrients. To do this, subtract the macronutrients from the brand linked and add in the macros for the brand you are using.

Each menu starts with a grocery list of the three recipes. There are exact measurements listed that you will need for the three recipes combined. There are some staple ingredients that you will notice are used throughout the recipes. Take note of the table below to reduce your ingredient cost by buying these items in larger quantities.

Recurring Grocery Items You Might Want to Buy in Bulk

Sprouted Oats
Soy milk
Nutritional yeast
Tahini
Lemon juice
Liquid aminos/soy sauce
Pure maple syrup
Vanilla protein powder
For a discount on protein powder head to my instagram @evannryan and hit the link in bio

Disclaimer

The recipes and macronutrients provided are not a tailored meal plan to you. They are built on the author's personal basis of a healthy and balanced approach to plant-based eating. If you require a professional meal plan to assist with medical or health issues please seek a registered health care professional.

The meal prep plan is simply a cookbook designed to make your life easier by helping you take the guesswork out of meal planning.

Many of the ingredients have a direct link where you can buy the author's favorite ingredients. Please note that the author does make a small commission on some of the linked items.

The author is a chef and not a registered dietician, so please take these recipes as they are meant to be, a healthy, sustainable way of eating from a chef's kitchen to yours.

Please note: all macros have been calculated with the intention of being as close to accurate as possible but may vary slightly.

Menu One

| 1566 CALS - 54G FAT - 167G CARBS - 88G PROTEIN |

BREAKFAST

The Best Tofu Scramble

The best Tofu Scramble, like seriously. The key is in warming the spices, using full fat coconut milk, and lots of creamy nutritional yeast. Add a handful of spinach to get your greens in, maybe pair it with some toast and you are good-to-go.

LUNCH

Creamy Cashew Slaw with Sweet Potatoes

Simple to come together with a pre-chopped salad bag, frozen veggies, and a simple blender dressing. This meal is a breeze to whip up.

DINNER

High Protein Tomato Soup

Tomato soup built for the high protein vegan! Red lentils kick the satiation factor way up in this chunky tomato soup recipe.

SNACK SUGGESTION FOR MENU ONE

Use up the other half of your coconut milk can with the Chia Protein Pudding

Macros below are the daily total if adding the Chia Pudding

| 2067 cals - 84g fat - 219g carbs - 110g protein |

GROCERY LIST - MENU ONE

<u>Pantry</u>

¼ cup olive oil
½ cup full fat coconut milk, canned
2 tsp <u>maple syrup</u>
6 cups <u>veggie broth</u> or vegetable bouillon cubes if preferred
3 tbsp tomato paste
2 tsp turmeric powder
1 tsp garlic powder
¼ cup + 1 tsp <u>nutritional yeast</u>
1 tsp onion powder
1 tbsp salt
1 tsp black pepper
½ cup raw cashews

<u>Produce</u>

2 yellow onions
2 cups fresh spinach
2 medium sweet potatoes
6 cups pre-chopped shredded cabbage mix
1 cup frozen corn
1 cup frozen english peas
5 cloves garlic
1 tbsp <u>lemon juice</u> or juice from a lemon
1 pint cherry tomatoes
1 package fresh basil

Protein

2 cups red lentils
2 bricks medium firm tofu
2 packages Smoked Fava Tofu
Carbs
4 Indian Life Tortillas
4 Sunflower Flax Sourdough
*This list does not include the ingredients for
Protein Chia Pudding*

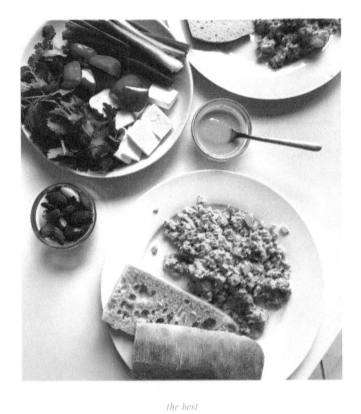

the best

TOFU
SCRAMBLE

| 343 CALS | 23G FAT | 7 CARBS | 23G PROTEIN |

The Best Tofu Scramble

Recipe makes 4 servings of Tofu Scramble
Macros per serving: 343 cals - 23g fat - 7g carbs -
29g protein

Complete the meal by wrapping in a tortilla for on
the go. The tortillas linked are less than 2g sugar
per serving, have a simple ingredients list, and are
always fresh and delicious.

Macros with tortillas listed:
| 633 cals - 30g fat - 56g carbs - 35g protein |

Ingredients:
1 tbsp olive oil
1 yellow onion, diced
2 tsp turmeric powder
1 tsp garlic powder
2 bricks medium firm tofu, crumbled by hand
½ cup full fat coconut milk, from a can
2 cups fresh spinach
¼ cup nutritional yeast
1 tsp salt
4 Indian Life Tortillas

Recipe:
1. Preheat a pan to medium heat, add oil,
coating the bottom
Add diced yellow onion and saute until softened,
3-4 minutes
2. Add turmeric powder and garlic powder
and warm through, 30 seconds

3. Add crumbled tofu and mix well, coating the tofu and coloring it yellow
4. Add coconut milk, fresh chopped spinach, and nutritional yeast

Mix everything well to combine and reduce heat to low

Cook until spinach is wilted and tofu is warmed through, 3 - 4 minutes

5. Turn off heat and season with salt
6. Plate and top with cracked pepper to activate the turmeric
7. If using a tortilla: gently roll scramble into 4 tortillas and store in the fridge

These wraps are great toasted in a panini grill, or pan fried on the stove in a small amount of oil or plant-based butter.

Increase the portion

Add veggie sausage to the wrap for up to 25g extra protein per serving

Add extra veggies, like bell peppers or kale for extra flavor with minimal calories

Add a serving of black beans for added fiber and protein

Add avocado for healthy fats and potassium

Add store bought salsa for extra flavor without the chopping

CASHEW
SLAW

254 CALS	8G FAT	26 CARBS	22G PROTEIN

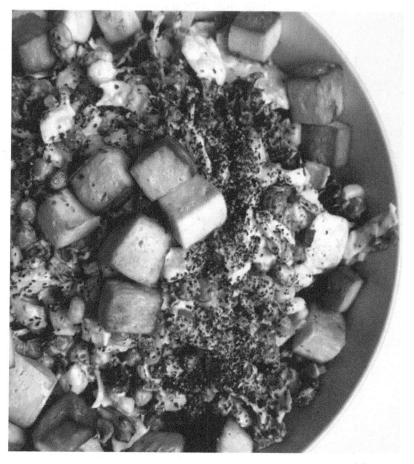

Creamy Cashew Slaw with Smoked Fava Tofu

Recipe makes 4 servings Cashew Slaw
Macros per serving: 254 cals - 8g fat - 26g carbs - 22g protein

Complete the meal with a side of sweet potatoes.

Macros for complete meal:
| 365 cals - 12g fat - 45g carbs - 24g protein |

Ingredients:
2 medium sweet potatoes, sliced into wedges
1 tbsp olive oil
1/2 tsp sea salt
1/4 tsp black pepper
Optional: add a pinch of chili powder to spice it up

Salad mix:
6 cups pre-chopped shredded cabbage
1 cup organic frozen corn
1 cup frozen english peas
2 package Smoked Fava Tofu

Cashew Dressing:
½ cup raw cashews
½ cup water
3 cloves garlic
2 tbsp lemon juice

2 tsp maple syrup
1 tsp onion powder
1 tsp nutritional yeast
1 tsp salt

Recipe:
1. Preheat oven to 350 F and line a baking tray with parchment paper
Toss your sweet potato wedges in oil, salt, pepper, and chili powder
Spread evenly across baking tray
Bake for 20-25 minutes or until cooked through, set aside
2. Cube your fava tofu and toss in olive oil and salt, bake for 12 minutes or until just slightly browning, set aside
3. Bring a small pot of water to a boil and add your frozen corn and frozen peas, allow to boil 3-4 minutes, drain and rinse with cold water, set aside
4. Add all your Cashew Dressing ingredients to a high speed blender and blend until smooth
5. Add all your salad ingredients to a bowl including dressing and toss to combine
6. Plate 4 salads each with a side of roasted sweet potatoes

Increase the portion

Wrap it up in a tortilla for higher carbs

Add 1-2 tbsp hemp seeds for additional protein and healthy fats

Bulk up the size with additional veggies

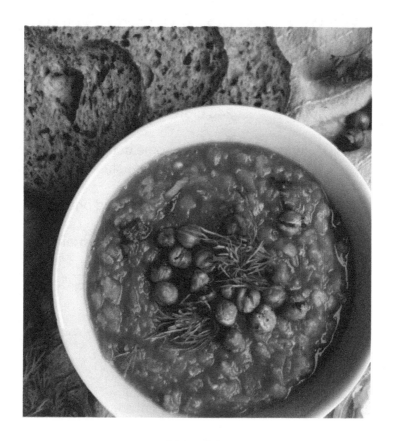

high protein

TOMATO
SOUP

438 CALS | 9G FAT | 66 CARBS | 24G PROTEIN

High Protein Tomato Soup

Recipe makes 4 servings of Tomato Soup
Macros per serving: 438 cals - 9g fat - 66g carbs -
24g protein

Complete the meal with some gut loving,
fermented sourdough toast.

Macros for one serving Tomato Soup and one slice
listed sourdough bread:
| 568 cals - 12g fat - 86g carbs - 29g protein |

Ingredients:
2 tbsp olive oil
1 yellow onion, diced
2 cloves garlic, diced
1 pint cherry tomato, halved
3 tbsp tomato paste
5-6 cups <u>veggie broth</u>
2 cups <u>red lentils</u>, rinsed
1 tsp sea salt
1 package fresh basil
4 <u>Sunflower Flax Sourdough</u>

Recipe:
1. Bring a pot to medium heat and add olive
oil, coating the bottom of the pan
Add diced onion, and saute until softened, 3-4
minutes
2. Add garlic and warm through, 1 minute

3. Add cherry tomatoes and cook until bursting, 4-5 minutes
4. Add tomato paste, veggie broth, red lentils, and salt
Mix everything well, and bring to a boil
5. Once boiling reduce heat to a simmer and cook until red lentils are cooked through, 20-25 minutes, stirring occasionally to make sure nothing is sticking to the bottom of the pan
6. Once ready to eat add fresh basil to each bowl and stir through
7. Enjoy with freshly toasted sourdough

Increase the portion

Buy pre-seasoned smokey tempeh and bake, add to top of soup as a crouton for additional protein and probiotics

Make a side salad or pair it with a vegan grilled cheese for added fats and carbs

CHIA
PUDDING

| 501 CALS | 30G FAT | 52 CARBS | 22G PROTEIN |

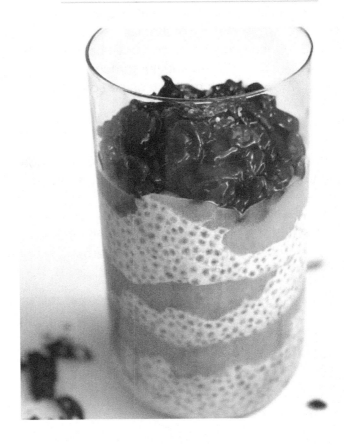

Protein Chia Pudding

Recipe makes 4 servings of Chia Pudding

Macros per serving:
| 501 cals - 30g fat - 52g carbs - 22g protein |

Ingredients:
¾ cup chia seeds
40g vanilla protein
1 cup soy milk
1 cup water
2 cup frozen mango
1 cup granola
½ Pomegranate Hazelnut Chocolate Bar

Recipe:
1. Add frozen mango to a small sauce pot with ½ cup water
2. Bring heat to medium low and cook until water has evaporated and mango is soft
3. Add mango to a blender and blend until smooth, set in the fridge to cool
4. In a mixing bowl add: chia seeds, vanilla protein, soy milk, and water, whisking everything to combine
5. Pour into two bowls and set in the fridge to form a pudding, 30 minutes or up to overnight
6. Melt chocolate bar in the microwave or over a double broiler, making sure to stir often so the chocolate doesn't burn

7. Add granola to melted chocolate and toss to coat in the chocolate
8. Once chia mixture has formed a pudding, top with mango puree and chocolate covered granola

Menu Two

| 1587 CALS - 62 G FAT - 141 G CARBS - 89 G PROTEIN |

BREAKFAST

Roasted Pesto Sandwich

This flavor packed sandwich tastes like something you paid too much for at a fancy coffee shop, but ten times more delicious and with way more hunger satiating protein.

LUNCH

Buffalo Chickpea Salad

Tender chickpea balls rolled in buffalo sauce, perfectly paired with a "cool down the heat" herby vinaigrette dressing.

DINNER

Mongolian "Beef" Noodles

Have you ever heard the term "fakeaway"? It's the healthier, homemade version of your favorite junky takeout meal. These saucy noodles hit all the notes with ginger and garlic, while absolutely smashing the protein with veggie grounds and legume noodles.

SNACK SUGGESTION FOR MENU TWO

With the additional brown rice flour and coconut sugar make the Cinnamon Sugar Protein Donuts

Macros below are the daily total if adding two Cinnamon Sugar Donuts
| 1845 cals - 74g fat - 171g carbs - 99g protein |

GROCERY LIST - MENU TWO

<u>Pantry</u>

¼ cup + 2 tbsp soy milk - will be used again in the next menu!
1/4 + 2 tbsp <u>Bragg Soy Sauce</u>
¼ cup + 2 tbsp <u>nutritional yeast</u>
1/4 tsp turmeric powder
2 tsp garlic powder
2 tbsp chili flakes
2 tbsp <u>buffalo style hot sauce</u>, or other favorite hot sauce
1 tbsp apple cider vinegar, or other preferred vinegar
1 tbsp salt
1 tsp black pepper
2 tbsp + 1 tsp extra virgin olive oil
1 tbsp <u>sesame oil</u>, can sub olive oil if preferred
⅓ cup <u>tahini</u>, used in many other recipes coming up!
1/4 cup walnuts
2 cup <u>veggie broth</u>

<u>Produce</u>

1 red bell pepper
4 cups broccoli florets
½ zucchini
3 cups spinach
1 tbsp <u>lemon juice</u> or juice from a lemon

2 cups purple cabbage, thinly sliced
1 cucumber
1 large carrot
1 bunch green onions
6 clove garlic
2 tbsp fresh dill
2 tbsp fresh parsley
2 inch fresh ginger
1 yellow onion

Protein

1 brick medium firm tofu
2 packages Chickapea Pasta shells
1 pack Gusta Foods veggie grounds
2 cups canned chickpeas
¼ cup aquafaba, brine from the can of chickpeas
(SAVE from canned chickpeas!)
Carbs
4 Almond Buns
½ cup brown rice, cooked - can buy microwave
rice packet if preferred

*This list does not include the ingredients for
Cinnamon Sugar Donuts*

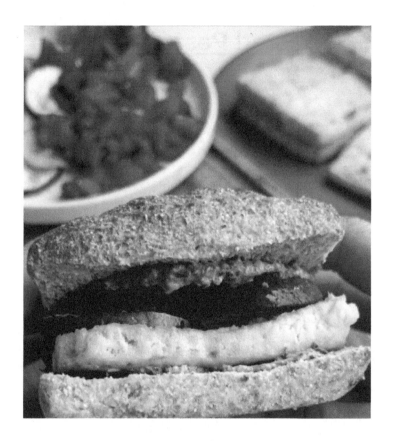

roasted

PESTO
SANDWICH

495 CALS | 35G FAT | 16G CARBS | 24G PROTEIN

Roasted Pesto Sandwich

Recipe makes 4 sandwiches

Macros per sandwich:
| 495 cals - 35g fat - 16g carbs - 24g protein |

Ingredients:
1 brick medium firm tofu
1 tbsp nutritional yeast
1/4 tsp turmeric powder
1 tsp garlic powder
½ salt
1 red bell pepper, diced
½ zucchini , sliced into thin rounds
2 tsp extra virgin olive oil
4 Almond Buns

Spinach Walnut Pesto:
3 cups spinach
1/4 cup walnuts
2 tbsp extra virgin olive oil
1 tbsp lemon juice
2 tsp nutritional yeast
1 clove garlic
½ tsp salt

Recipe:
1. Preheat oven to 350 F and line a baking tray
with parchment paper

2. Slice your tofu into 4 squares and add to baking tray
Drizzle a tsp of olive oil over squares and season with 1 tbsp nutritional yeast, turmeric powder, garlic powder, and salt, use your hands to coat the squares evenly

3. Bake for 12-15 minutes or until browned, flip, and bake for another 3-4 minutes or until browned on the second side remove from oven and set aside

4. To another baking tray add diced bell peppers, and zucchini rounds and season with 1 tsp oil and salt

5. Bake for 15 minutes or until browned, set aside

6. Make your pesto: add everything to a high speed blender and blend until smooth

7. Slice your buns and coat each side with pesto, layer your baked tofu, peppers, and zucchini

8. Enjoy cold, warm in a panini grill, lightly fry them on the stove top like a grilled cheese, or microwave for 1-2 minutes

Increase the portion

Make a side of roasted potatoes for additional carbs

Add some pre-seasoned tempeh bacon to boost
protein
Make it a wrap and add more of everything!

buffalo

CHICKPEA
SALAD

490 CALS | 15G FAT | 69G CARBS | 21G PROTEIN

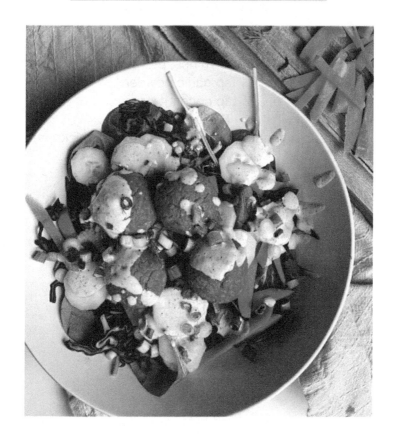

Buffalo Chickpea Salad

Makes 4 servings

Macros per salad:
| 490 cals - 15g fat - 69g carbs - 21g protein |

Ingredients, Buffalo Chickpea Balls:
2 cups canned chickpeas
¼ cup nutritional yeast
2 tbsp buffalo style hot sauce
½ cup brown rice, pre-cooked*
1 tsp garlic powder
½ tsp coconut sugar
Big pinch salt
¼ cup aquafaba, brine from the can of chickpeas
½ cup brown rice flour

Ingredients, Salad:
2 cups purple cabbage, thinly sliced
1 cucumber, sliced
1 large carrot, peeled and chopped
1 bunch green onions, chopped

Creamy Herb Dressing:
⅓ cup tahini
1 tbsp apple cider vinegar
2 tbsp fresh dill
2 tbsp fresh parsley
2 cloves garlic
1 tsp black pepper
½ tsp salt
¼ cup + 2 tbsp soy milk

Recipe, Buffalo Chickpea Balls:

1. Pre-cook your brown rice, set aside
NOTE: You can buy microwave rice packets in small quantities, or you can cook a batch at home, cool and freeze the remainder for up to one month

2. Preheat oven to 425 F and line a baking tray with parchment paper

3. To a high speed blender or food processor add everything, except the brown rice flour, and blend until a smooth batter forms

4. Pour the batter into a mixing bowl and gently fold in brown rice flour until just incorporated

5. Using an ice cream scoop or a large spoon gently form 14 balls, placing them onto the baking tray

6. Bake for 12-15 minutes, or until slightly cracking and browned on the bottoms

7. Allow to sit 5 minutes before gently tossing them in hot sauce

Salad:

1. Prepare your veggies and set aside

Creamy Herb Dressing:

1. Add everything to a high speed blender and blend until smooth

Plate your salad:

1. Add you dressing to the bottom of four containers

2. Add 1/4 of the salad mix to each

3. Divide the chickpea balls evenly across the four containers

4. Seal and refrigerate until ready to eat

<u>*Increase the portion*</u>

Add additional brown rice to the bowl

Add a serving of edamame beans or veggie sausage to increase protein

Add avocado for additional healthy fats

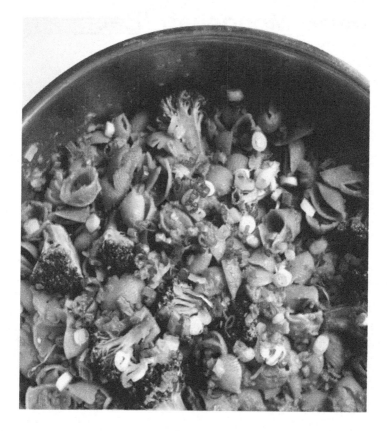

mongolian

'BEEF'
NOODLES

602 CALS | 12G FAT | 56G CARBS | 44G PROTEIN

Mongolian "Beef" Noodles

Recipe makes 4 servings

Macros per serving:
| 602 cals - 12g fat - 56g carbs - 44g protein |

Ingredients:
2 packages Chickapea Pasta shells
1 tbsp sesame oil
2 inch fresh ginger, chopped
3 cloves garlic, chopped
1 yellow onion
1 pack veggie grounds
2 cup veggie broth
4 cups broccoli florets
1/4 + 2 tbsp Bragg Soy Sauce
1/4 cup coconut sugar
2 tbsp chili flakes

Recipe:

1. Prepare your noodles according to package directions, reserve 1/2 cup pasta water

2. Meanwhile, preheat a pan to medium heat and add sesame oil - coating the pan

3. To the pan add chopped ginger, garlic and onion with a touch of salt and saute, 2-3 minutes

4. Add veggie grounds and toss through the onions,garlic,ginger mix

5. Add veggie broth and broccoli

6. Mix and allow to cook another 3-4 minutes or until veggie grounds and broccoli are mostly cooked

7. Add cooked pasta, ¼ reserved pasta water and soy sauce, coconut sugar, and chili flakes, stirring everything together well

8. Remove from heat and allow everything to marry, 2-3 minutes

9. Top with green onion if desired

Increase the portion
Add black beans for additional protein and fiber

cinnamon

SUGAR
DONUTS

129 CALS	6G FAT	15G CARBS	5G PROTEIN

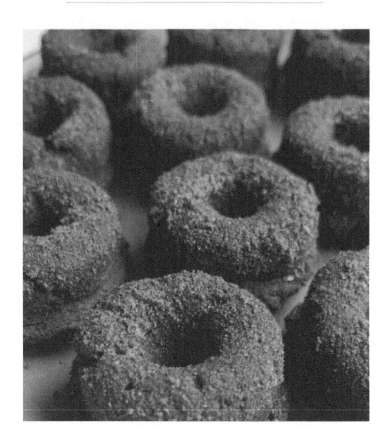

Cinnamon Sugar Baked Mini Donuts

Recipe makes 12 donuts

Macros per donut:
| 129 cals - 6g fat - 15g carbs - 5g protein |

Ingredients:
1 banana
1/3 cup + 2 tbsp coconut milk
1/4 cup vegan butter
1/2 cup coconut sugar
3/4 cup oat flour
1/2 cup vanilla protein
2 tsp ceylon cinnamon
1 tsp baking powder
1/2 tsp baking soda

Coating:
2 tbsp melted vegan butter
1 tbsp ceylon cinnamon
2 tbsp coconut sugar

Recipe:
1. Preheat oven to 350 F

2. Grease a mini donut pan (if you don't have one just use muffin liners and add 1-2 minutes to bake time)

3. Add the banana and coconut milk to a blender and blend until smooth, set aside

4. Cream butter and coconut sugar together

5. Add banana/coconut milk mixture to creamed butter/coconut sugar mixture and fold together with a spatula

6. Add all the dry ingredients: oat flour, vanilla protein, cinnamon, baking powder and baking soda to the wet ingredients

7. Fold everything together until just incorporated

8. Add batter to donut pan with a spoon, smoothing over the tops of each

9. Bake for 9-10 minutes or until they've risen, browned around the edges and slightly cracked on the tops

10. Allow to cool completely before removing from pan

11. Add melted butter to a bowl and toss the cooled donuts in, coating them in a thin layer of butter

12. Add cinnamon and sugar to another small bowl and toss the buttered donuts in to coat completely

Menu Three

BREAKFAST

Cake Batter Protein Oats

A birthday cake that feeds the body and soul! Super rich and creamy, topped with crumbly cookie bits and sprinkles, this bowl of oats is as fun to eat as it is healthy.

LUNCH

White Bean Chopped Salad

Simple and minimal chopping, this salad is well rounded for the perfect grab and go meal prep.

DINNER

Peanut Satay Bowl

The flavor packed fitness meal you're going to be excited to eat! Well seasoned tempeh, roasted yams, and bright green beans are the perfect pairing for a spicy peanut sauce.
Hot tip: yams and peanut butter were made for eachother.

SNACK SUGGESTION FOR MENU THREE

With such a low calorie count for the overall menu, this is the perfect week to make the vegan cream cheese recipe and add a bagel or two to your day with a savory dairy free cream cheese you're going to love!

Macros below are the daily total if adding one serving of Tofu Cream Cheese with one bagel

| 1688 cals - 57g fat - 185g carbs - 97g protein |

GROCERY LIST - MENU THREE

<u>Pantry</u>

2 cups sprouted oats
2 1/2 cups soy milk
60g vanilla pea protein
2 cup canned cannellini beans
½ cup + 2 tbsp canned coconut milk
1/4 cup hemp seeds
1/3 cup almonds
¼ cup + 2 tbsp peanut butter powder
4 Coco D'lish cookie - can sub another cookie if preferred
1/4 cup rice vinegar
3 tbsp olive oil
1 tbsp + 2 tsp maple syrup
2 tbsp chili flakes
1/2 tsp salt
¼ cup + 2 tsp soy sauce
1 tbsp curry powder

<u>Protein</u>

1 package veggie grounds
2 bricks plain tempeh
Produce
1 red onion
1/2 cup parsley
2 cups yams
2 cloves garlic

1 lime
2 cups green beans

Other

1 cup plain vegan yogurt - yogurt is used again in
the next menu!
1 tbsp vanilla extract
2-3 tbsp vegan sprinkles

*This list does not include ingredients for the Vegan
Cream Cheese recipe*

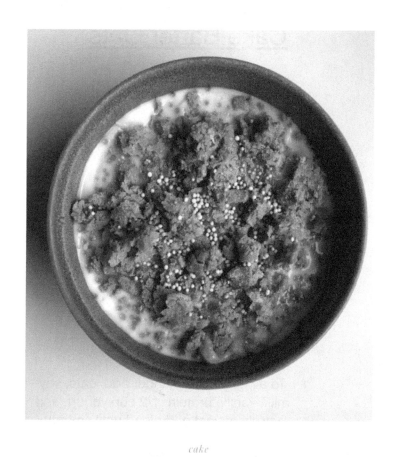

cake

BATTER
OATS

| 440 CALS | 13G FAT | 48 CARBS | 26G PROTEIN |

Cake Batter Oats

Recipe makes 4 servings

Macros per serving:
| 440 cals - 13g fat - 48g carbs - 26g protein |

Ingredients:
2 cups sprouted oats
2 1/2 cups soy milk
60g vanilla pea protein
1/2 cup plain vegan yogurt + 1/2 cup more for the top
1 tbsp vanilla extract
2-3 tbsp vegan sprinkles
4 Coco D'lish cookie crumbled

Recipe:
1. To a high speed blender add: oats, soy milk, vanilla protein, 1/2 cup yogurt, and vanilla extract and blend until smooth

2. Pour into a bowl or container and set in the fridge until firm, 1-2 hrs or overnight

3. Add 2 tbsp of yogurt to the top of each bowl of oats smoothing it with a spoon

4. Cover in sprinkles and a crumbled cookie

Increase the portion

Use a protein cookie, like Lenny & Larry's for the top!

triple protein

CHOPPED
SALAD

| 407 CALS | 13G FAT | 37 CARBS | 27G PROTEIN |

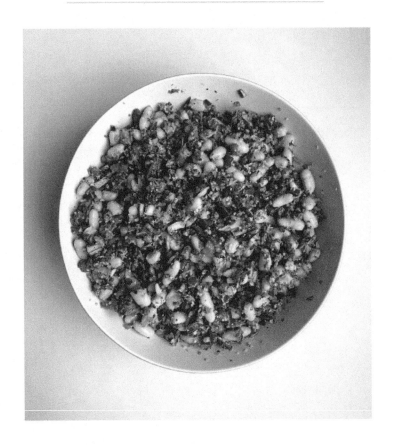

White Bean Chopped Salad

Recipe makes 4 servings

Macros per serving:
| 407 cals - 13g fat - 37g carbs -27g protein |

Ingredients:
2 cup canned cannellini beans, drained and rinsed
1 package veggie grounds
1/3 cup almonds, chopped
1/4 cup hemp seeds
1 red onion, diced
1/2 cup parsley, chopped
1/4 cup rice vinegar
2 tbsp olive oil
2 tsp maple syrup
1 tbsp chili flakes
1/2 tsp salt

Recipe:
1. Preheat oven to 350 F and line a baking tray with parchment paper

2. Spread your veggie grounds across baking tray and bake for 10-15 minutes, or until browned, set aside

3. Drain and rinse your beans and add to a large mixing bowl

4. Add to mixing bowl: cooked grounds, almonds, hemp seeds, red onions, parsley

5. To a small bowl add: rice vinegar, olive oil, maple syrup, chili flakes, and salt, whisk to combine

6. Pour dressing over salad and toss well

7. Plate into 4 containers, seal, and place in the fridge until ready to eat

Increase the portion

Add 1-2 cups of rice or quinoa for additional carbs

Bulk it up with a bed of mixed greens or more herbs for minimal calories

Add cold legume noodles for additional protein and carbs
Wrap it up for more carbs and calories

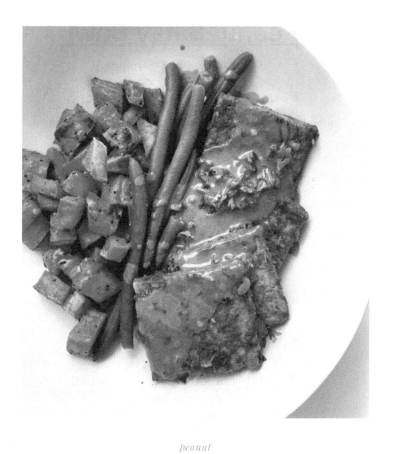

peanut

SATAY
BOWL

474 CALS | 18G FAT | 48 CARBS | 29G PROTEIN

Peanut Satay Bowl

Recipe makes 4 servings

Macros per serving:
| 474 cals - 18g fat - 48g carbs - 29g protein |

Ingredients:
2 cups yams, cubed
1 tbsp olive oil
2 bricks plain tempeh
¼ cup soy sauce
1 tbsp curry powder
½ cup full fat coconut milk, canned
2 cloves garlic, minced

Peanut Sauce:
¼ cup + 2 tbsp peanut butter powder
3 tbsp water
2 tbsp full fat coconut milk, canned
2 tsp soy sauce
2 tsp lime juice
1 tbsp maple syrup
1 tbsp chili flakes
2 cups green beans

Recipe:
1. Preheat oven to 350 F and line baking tray with parchment paper

2. Prepare your yams and toss in olive oil, salt, and pepper

3. Spread seasoned yams across baking tray and bake for
20-25 minutes or until lightly browned around the edges and cooked through, set aside

4. Prepare your tempeh by slicing 8 thin squares

5. To a small bowl add soy sauce, curry powder, coconut milk, and minced garlic cloves, whisk to combine

6. Heat a frying pan to medium heat and add half the sauce
and half the tempeh

7. Allow to cook for 4-5 minutes or until sauce has reduced by half

8. Flip the tempeh and cook until the sauce has been
completely absorbed by the tempeh, continuing to cook until you have a nice crisp browning on the tempeh

9. Remove and repeat with remaining sauce and tempeh

10. To make the peanut sauce add everything to a bowl and whisk well to combine
If too thick, add more water, too thin, add more peanut butter powder

11. For the green beans, bring a small pot of water to a boil
Add the green beans once boiling, allowing to cook for 4 minutes

12. Drain and immediately rinse with cold water or place in an ice bath to stop from cooking further

13.. Plate 1/4 of each recipe into four containers, and drizzle with peanut sauce

Increase the portion

Make more protein packed peanut sauce

Add another side veggie to the mix, like broccoli

Up the serving of yams for more complex carbs

Add edamame beans or additional tempeh for more protein

tofu

CREAM
CHEESE

| 107 CALS | 7G FAT | 6G CARBS | 9G PROTEIN |

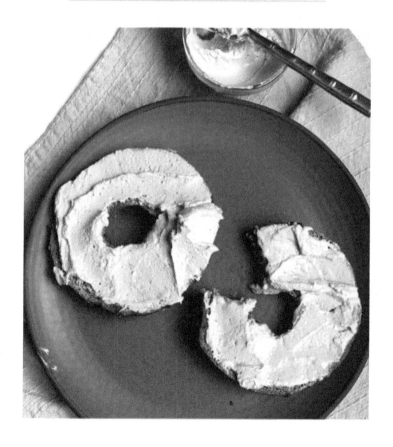

Tofu Cream Cheese

Recipe makes 6 large servings

Macros per serving of Cream Cheese:
| 107 cals - 7g fat - 6g carbs - 9g protein |

Ingredients:
1 brick medium firm tofu
1/4 cup walnuts
1 tsp salt
1 tbsp maple syrup
1 tbsp apple cider vinegar
2 tsp lemon juice
1 tsp garlic powder

6 bagels

Recipe:
1. Add everything to a food processor or high speed blender and blend until smooth, at least 4 minutes but keep in mind the longer you blend the smoother it gets!

Menu Four

| 1441 CALS - 55 G FAT - 160G CARBS - 102 G PROTEIN |

BREAKFAST

Peanut Butter Cup Oats

Like a breakfast peanut butter cup but creamier, lighter and way higher in protein!

LUNCH

Loaded Caesar Salad

If you haven't had a dairy free caesar salad you love yet, then you're about to. This one packs a punch with a tahini rich dressing, complex carbs from roasted yams, and a simple roasted protein. This salad will keep you full for hours.

DINNER

Tahini Noodle Bowl

Double the texture with creamy noodles and crispy roasted veggies. This simple meal has its protein disguised in the shape of pasta and a cream sauce.

SNACK SUGGESTION FOR MENU FOUR

Put that peanut butter powder to use and make the high protein peanut butter cake!
To note: If you are allergic to peanuts, simply substitute your favorite nut or seed butter in the Peanut Butter Cup Oats and try a high protein dip from the bonus pages!

Macros below are the daily total if adding two slices of Peanut Butter Snack Cake

| 1781 cals - 61g fat - 210g carbs - 118g protein |

GROCERY LIST - MENU FOUR

<u>Pantry</u>

2 cup sprouted oats
2/3 cup tahini
3 tbsp lemon juice
2 tbsp apple cider vinegar
2 tbsp dijon mustard
2 cups soy milk
¼ cup olive oil
½ tsp garlic powder
½ tsp paprika
1 tsp salt
2 tsp black pepper
1 tbsp <u>nutritional yeast</u>
1 tbsp capers
¼ cup walnuts
2 tbsp soy sauce
1 tbsp maple syrup
60g scoop vanilla protein
1 tbsp + 1 tsp maca powder, optional
1/4 cup <u>peanut butter powder</u>
4 squares melted chocolate
1 <u>no whey chocolate pea'not' butter cup</u>, optional

<u>Produce</u>

2 medium yams
8 cups lacinato kale, rough chopped
2 cups purple cabbage, chopped

2 cups savoy cabbage, chopped
2 cups kale
1 inch fresh ginger
5 cloves garlic

Protein

2 brick Smoked Fava Tofu
227g box of legume noodles
1 tbsp vegan yogurt
*Grocery list does not include ingredients for
Peanut Butter Cake*

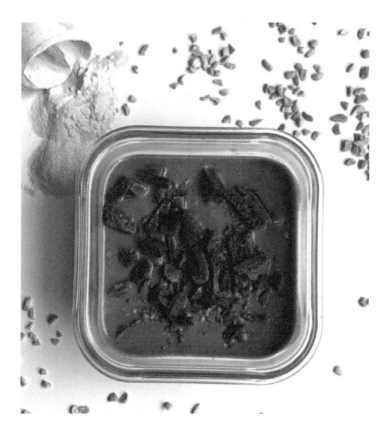

peanut

BUTTER CUP
OATS

| 435 CALS | 14G FAT | 44G CARBS | 30G PROTEIN |

Peanut Butter Cup Protein Oats

Recipe makes 4 servings

Macros per serving:
| 435 cals - 14g fat - 44g carbs - 30g protein |

Recipe note: Peanut butter powder is the defatted version of regular peanut butter. If you don't have this on hand you can substitute it for half the amount of regular peanut butter, but please note the macros will vary slightly.

Ingredients:
2 cup sprouted oats
60g scoop vanilla protein
1 tbsp + 1 tsp maca powder
1/4 cup peanut butter powder
2 cups soy milk
1 cup water

Topping:
¼ cup thick vegan yogurt
16 squares melted chocolate

Recipe:
1. To a blender add: oats, vanilla protein, maca powder, peanut butter powder, soy milk, and water, blend until smooth

2. Pour into four containers and place in the fridge to firm slightly, 15 minutes

3. Topping: melt chocolate and whisk into yogurt, pour over oats and place back in the fridge overnight to set

4. Option to add a chopped no whey chocolate peanut butter cup to the top

Increase the portion

Double down on the oats! This recipe calls for a 1/2 cup serving of oats, but you might just need a full cup! Just make sure to also increase your liquids.

Add a banana, either to the blender mix, or slices on top for additional carbs and fiber

Add an extra tablespoon of peanut butter to the top for added fats and 5g more protein

loaded

CAESAR
SALAD

438 CALS | 19G FAT | 48G CARBS | 39G PROTEIN

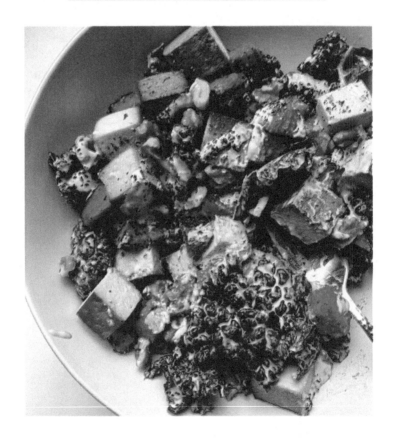

Loaded Caesar Salad

Recipe makes 4 servings

Macros per serving:
| 438 cals - 19g fat - 48g carbs - 39g protein |

Ingredients:
2 medium yams, cubed
2 tbsp olive oil
½ tsp garlic powder
½ tsp paprika
¼ tsp salt
2 brick Smoked Fava Tofua

Dressing:
⅓ cup tahini
2 tbsp lemon juice
2 tbsp apple cider vinegar
2 tbsp dijon mustard
1 tbsp nutritional yeast
4 cloves garlic
1 tbsp capers with the juice
2 tsp black pepper
½ tsp salt
½ cup water

Salad mix:
8 cups lacinato kale, rough chopped
¼ cup walnuts

Recipe:

1. Preheat oven to 375 F and line a baking tray with parchment paper, set aside

2. To a mixing bowl add: cubed yams, olive oil, garlic powder, paprika, and salt, tossing to combine

3. Spread evenly across baking tray and bake for 20-25 minutes or until browned and cooked through, set aside

4. Cube your fava tofu and spread evenly across a baking tray

5. Bake for 12 minutes or until lightly browned, set aside

6. To a high speed blender or food processor add all your dressing ingredients and blend until super smooth
7. Add prepared kale to a mixing bowl and coat in the dressing, massaging it in gently

8. Plate into four containers and top each with ¼ of the baked yams, and ½ brick baked fava tofu

9. Top with walnuts, seal and refrigerate until ready to eat

Increase the portion

Double the yams for more complex carbohydrates

Wrap it up in a tortilla for a more filling meal

Add pumpkin seeds to boost nutrition and healthy fats

Top with more nutritional yeast for an additional 3g protein per tablespoon and a nice cheesy flavour

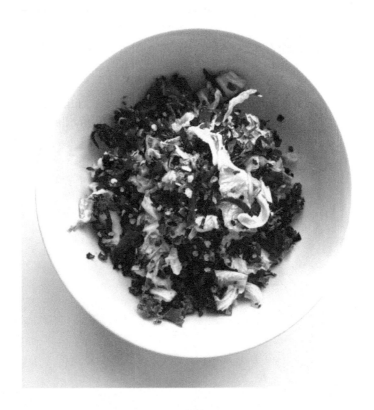

tahini

NOODLE
BOWL

568 CALS | 22G FAT | 68G CARBS | 33G PROTEIN

Tahini Noodle Bowl

Recipe makes 4 servings

Macros per serving:
| 568 cals - 22g fat - 68g carbs - 33g protein |

Ingredients:
227g box of legume noodles
2 cups purple cabbage, chopped
2 cups savoy cabbage, chopped
2 cups kale
2 tbsp extra virgin olive oil

Sauce:
⅓ cup tahini
1 tbsp lemon juice
1 clove garlic
1 inch ginger, peeled and rough chopped
2 tbsp soy sauce
1 tbsp maple syrup
⅓ cup water

Recipe:
1. Preheat the oven to 375 F and line a baking tray with parchment paper

2. Toss just the purple cabbage in 1 tbsp oil and a pinch of salt

3. Spread purple cabbage across baking tray and bake for 10 minutes

4. Remove from oven

5. Toss savoy cabbage in 1/2 tbsp oil and a pinch of salt and add to the purple cabbage baking tray, bake another 5-10 minutes

6. Toss the kale in the remaining 1/2 tbsp oil and add to the baking tray, bake everything a final 5 minutes

7. Bring a small pot of water to a boil

8. Once boiling add pasta and cook according to package directions

9. Just prior to draining, remove ½ cup boiling liquids, set aside

10. Strain the pasta and add back to the pot

11. Place the pot back on the hot element, with the heat off

12. To the pot add the sauce, noodles and reserved boiling liquids, mix well to combine

13. Allow sauce and noodles to marry, 4-5 minutes

14. Plate into four containers and top with roasted vegetables

Increase the portion

Add an additional protein source like veggie
crumbles or sausage

Add more roasted veggies for a bigger meal

Add pumpkin seeds or hemp hearts for additional
healthy fats & protein

peanut butter

SNACK
CAKE

| 170 CALS | 3G FAT | 25G CARBS | 8G PROTEIN |

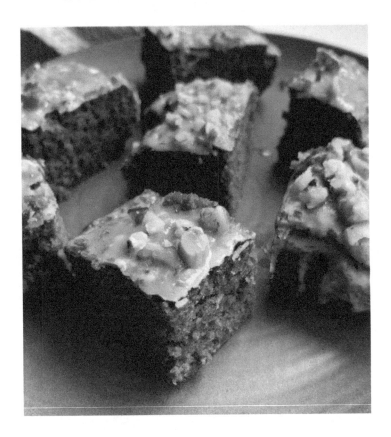

Peanut Butter Snack Cake

Makes 8 squares

Macros per piece:
170 cals - 3g fat - 25g carbs - 8g protein

Ingredients:
1 banana
1/3 cup soy milk
¼ cup plain vegan yogurt
½ cup coconut sugar
¾ cup peanut butter powder
½ cup gluten free flour
1 tsp baking powder
½ tsp baking soda
Pinch salt

Icing:
¼ cup icing sugar
1 tbsp peanut butter powder
1-2 tbsp soy milk

Recipe:
1. Preheat oven to 350 F and prepare a loaf pan with parchment paper or grease with oil or dairy free butter

2. To a high speed blender add: banana, soy milk, yogurt, and coconut sugar, blend until smooth

3. To a small mixing bowl sift: peanut butter powder, gluten free flour, baking powder, baking soda, and salt

4. Whisk to combine

5. Add wet ingredients to dry and mix together until just incorporated

6. Pour into prepared baking dish, smoothing the top with a spoon or spatula

7. Bake for 12- 15 minutes or until the center is puffed and the edges are lightly cracking

8. Allow to cool before removing from tray

9. For icing add everything together and mix well

10. Pour over cooled loaf, allowing it to drip down the sides
11. Top with crushed nuts if desired!

Menu Five

| 1676 CALS - 75 G FAT - 195 G CARBS - 93 G PROTEIN |

BREAKFAST

Eggless Quiche

A one pan meal that's packed with all your favorite breakfast foods. To make it weekend special on a weekday we've added a creamy sauce to drizzle on this hot pie.

LUNCH

Tempeh Sushi Bowl

A no roll sushi that hits all the fresh notes. Gut healthy fermented tempeh marinated in a sweet soy glaze, mixed with crisp cucumbers, sticky rice, and a tangy mayo sauce.

DINNER

Creamy Garlic White Beans

This meal is comfort in a bowl. A rich cream sauce filled with fiber rich cannellini beans and sausage, paired with roasted potato wedges. This meal prep bowl is like a warm hug after a long day.

SNACK SUGGESTION FOR MENU FIVE

Use any extra tahini and make the Peppermint Cacao Protein Bars!

Macros below are the daily total if adding one Peppermint Cacao Bar

1876 cals - 83g fat - 204g carbs - 102g protein

GROCERY LIST - MENU FIVE

<u>Pantry</u>

1 cup chickpea flour
2 tbsp hemp seeds
2 cups canned cannellini beans
3 tbsp tahini
2 cups white sticky rice
¼ cup soy sauce
2 tbsp + ½ tbsp maple syrup
1 ½ tbsp rice vinegar
1 ½ tbsp sesame oil
2 tbsp olive oil
2 tsp avocado oil, or other neutral cooking oil
¼ cup + 2 tbsp nutritional yeast
1 tbsp paprika
¼ tsp chili powder, or 1 tsp sriracha
1 tsp garlic powder
1 tsp baking powder
2 tbsp herb de provence, or any herb mix you like!
3 tbsp lemon juice
1 ½ cups coconut milk
½ cup veggie soup broth

<u>Protein</u>

2 bricks tempeh
1 1/2 cups edamame beans
2 veggie sausage
1 - 340g package veggie grounds

Produce
2 yukon potatoes
4 russet potatoes
20 brown mushrooms
4 persian cucumbers
2 jalapenos
1 cup cauliflower
1 cup kale
2 cups yams
2 cups cherry tomatoes
4 cloves garlic
2 cups frozen peas

Other

¼ cup vegan mayo

Grocery list does not include ingredients for Peppermint Cacao Bars

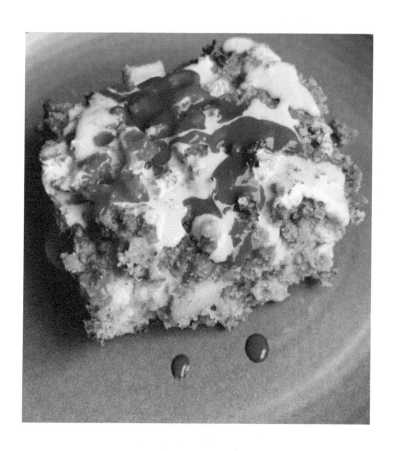

EGGLESS QUICHE

| 401 CALS | 16G FAT | 43G CARBS | 29G PROTEIN |

Eggless Quiche

Recipe makes 4 servings

Macros per serving with sauce:
| 401 cals - 16g fat - 43g carbs - 29g protein |

Ingredients:
1 cup chickpea flour
¼ cup nutritional yeast
1 tbsp paprika
1 tsp garlic powder
1 tsp baking powder
1 tsp salt
2 yukon potatoes, chopped
20 brown mushrooms, halved
1 - 340g package veggie grounds
1 cup cauliflower, chopped
1 cup kale, chopped

Sauce:
3 tbsp tahini
2 tbsp hemp seeds
2 tbsp nutritional yeast
1/4 tsp salt
2-3 tbsp water

Recipe:
1. Preheat oven to 375 F and line a 8x8 inch
    pan with parchment paper, or grease pan
    with vegan butter or oil, set aside

2. In a large mixing bowl add: chickpea flour, nutritional yeast, paprika, garlic powder, baking powder, and salt, whisking to combine

3. Add 1 ½ cups water to flour mixture and whisk to combine, set aside

4. Prepare your veggies, making sure to chop your potatoes small so they cook through

5. Add all your prepared veggies and veggie grounds to the wet mixture and mix through

6. Pour into baking pan and press down evenly

7. Bake in the oven for 30-35 minutes or until browned on top and cooked through

8. Allow to cool slightly before slicing into 4 pieces

Sauce:

1. Add all your ingredients to a high speed blender and blend until smooth

If sauce is too thick, add more water 1 tbsp at a time

Increase the portion

Add an additional protein source to the quiche mix, like soft tofu

Have a side of toast for additional carbs

Add a side of avocado for additional healthy fats

tempeh

SUSHI
BOWL

648 CALS | 25G FAT | 72G CARBS | 28G PROTEIN

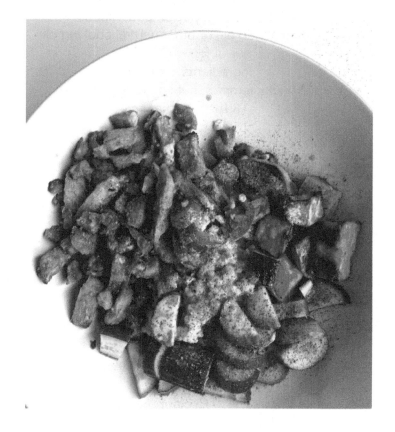

Tempeh Sushi Bowl Prep

Recipe makes 4 servings

Macros per serving:
| 648 cals - 25g fat - 72g carbs - 28g protein |

Ingredients:
2 cups <u>white sticky rice</u>, prepared
2 cups yams, peeled and cubed
2 tsp avocado oil, or other neutral cooking oil

Ingredients, Tempeh:
2 bricks tempeh, cut into rough pieces
3 tbsp <u>soy sauce</u>
1 ½ tbsp <u>sesame oil</u>
2 tbsp <u>maple syrup</u>

Tangy Mayo:
¼ cup vegan mayo
1 ½ tbsp <u>rice vinegar</u>
1 tbsp <u>soy sauce</u>
½ tbsp <u>maple syrup</u>
¼ tsp chili powder, or 1 tsp sriracha

Sushi Bowl add-ins:
1 1/2 cups edamame beans
4 persian cucumbers, sliced
2 jalapenos, chopped thin

Recipe:
1. Make white sticky rice according to package directions and set aside

2.   Preheat oven to 375 F and line a baking tray
with parchment paper

3.   Peel and chop your yams into cubes and
toss in 2 tsp oil and a pinch of salt

4.   Spread evenly across baking tray and bake
for 20-23 minutes or until browned and
cooked through, set aside

5.   Line a baking tray with parchment paper,
set aside

6.   Prepare tempeh by chopping into
mismatched pieces

7.   Add tempeh pieces to a bowl and toss with
soy sauce, sesame oil, and maple syrup

8.   Spread evenly across baking tray and bake
for 14-16
minutes or until the biggest pieces are browned

9. Make Tangy Mayo sauce by adding everything
to a bowl and whisking to combine

10. Prepare additional add-ins: edamame,
cucumber, jalapenos

9. Plate everything into 4 containers and drizzle
with tangy mayo, enjoy with an extra side of soy
sauce if desired

Increased portion

Double the edamame for more protein

Add more fresh veggies to boost the portion with
minimal extra calories

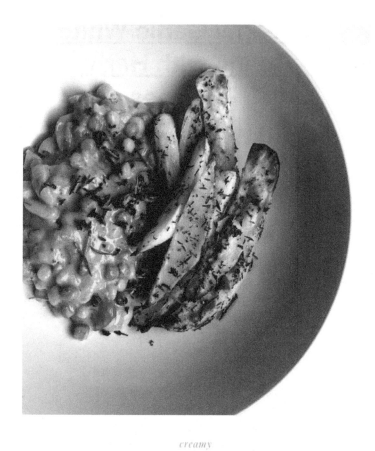

creamy

GARLIC
WHITE BEANS

627 CALS | 34G FAT | 80G CARBS | 36G PROTEIN

Creamy Garlic White Beans with Herby Potatoes

Recipe makes 4 servings

Macros per serving:
| 627 cals - 34g fat - 80g carbs - 36g protein |

Ingredients, Potatoes:
4 russet potatoes, peeled and cut into wedges
3 tbsp lemon juice
2 tbsp olive oil
2 tbsp herb de provence, or any herb mix you like!
½ tsp sea salt
½ tsp black pepper

2 veggie sausage

Cream Sauce:
4 cloves garlic, chopped
1 ½ cups coconut milk
½ cup veggie broth
2 cups cherry tomatoes
1 tsp salt
1 tsp black pepper
2 cups canned cannellini beans, drained and rinsed
2 cups frozen peas

Recipe:

1. Preheat oven to 375 F and line a baking tray with parchment paper

2. Prep potatoes and season, spread evenly across baking tray

3. Bake potatoes for 20 minutes, then remove from oven and flip each potato and add your veggie sausages to the baking tray

4. Bake the sausages and potatoes for 10-12 minutes more

5. Once done, remove from oven and rough chop your cooked sausages, set aside

Cream Sauce
1. To a pot add: garlic, coconut milk, broth, cherry tomatoes, salt, and pepper

2. Bring to boil then reduce heat to simmer and cook, 15 minutes, allowing sauce to reduce by half

3. Add chopped sausages and cannellini beans to pot and allow to heat through, 5 minutes

4. Add frozen peas and let cook another 2-3 minutes or until heated through

5. Remove from heat and allow to sit another 10-15 minutes - sauce will thicken as it sits

6. Plate into 4 containers with roasted potatoes

<u>*Increase the portion*</u>

Add extra veggies like broccoli or asparagus

Add additional portions of sausages or beans for additional protein

peppermint

CACAO
BARS

200 CALS | 8G FAT | 9G CARBS | 9G PROTEIN

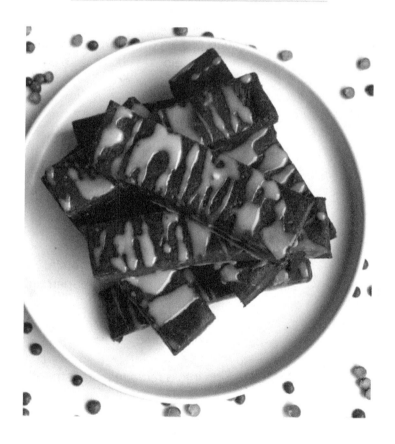

Peppermint Cacao Bars

Recipe makes 12 bars

Macros per bar:
| 200 cals - 8g fat - 9g carbs - 9g protein |

Ingredients:
1 cup tahini
1 cup probiotic cacao protein powder or chocolate protein
¼ cup cocoa powder
½ cup almond flour
⅓ cup maple syrup
1 tbsp peppermint extract

3-4 tbsp Icing sugar
2 tsp water or dairy free milk
Tiny drop of green food coloring, optional

Recipe:
1. To a mixing bowl add: tahini, protein, almond flour, maple syrup, and peppermint extract

2. Mix well forming a dough

3. Spread dough into a rectangle and smooth

4. Add to the freezer to firm, 30 minutes- 1 hr

5. Remove from freezer and cut into bars 8 bars

6. Icing glaze: add icing sugar, water or milk, and food coloring to a small bowl and mix until smooth

7. Drizzle over bars and allow icing to set, 10 minutes

8. Best eaten straight from the fridge or freezer!

BONUS: Three High Protein Dips

High Protein Hummus

Creamy, rich, hummus with the bonus of vitamin rich pumpkin seed protein powder. The pumpkin seed powder blends in seamlessly and adds nutrients and protein.

Edamame and Pea Dip

Get greens and protein in at snack time. Velvety, smooth and perfect for any time of day.

High Protein Tahini Dip

Light and creamy, this dip is also a great salad dressing or bowl topper!

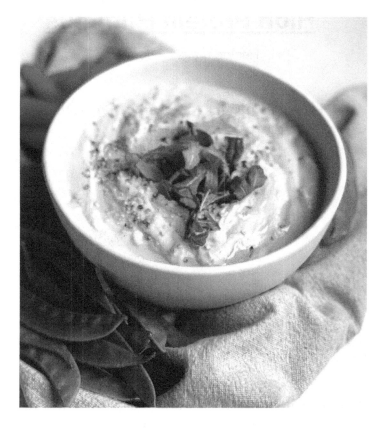

high

PROTEIN
HUMMUS

| 138 CALS | 9G FAT | 11G CARBS | 6G PROTEIN |

High Protein Hummus

Recipe makes 8 servings

Macros per serving:
| 138 cals - 9g fat - 11g carbs - 6g protein |

Ingredients:
2 cups chickpeas
¼ cup tahini
3 cloves garlic
2 tbsp lemon juice
25g scoop pumpkin seed protein
2 tbsp extra virgin olive oil
1 tsp salt
½ cup water

Recipe:
Add everything to high speed blender and blend
until super smooth, the longer you blend the
smoother it becomes
Recipe note: add more water 1 tbsp at a time if you
prefer a thinner consistency

Enjoy with whole wheat pita, crackers, or chopped
vegetables

Increase the portion

Make a veggie sandwich smothered in hummus

Enjoy with smoked tofu for additional protein and
no cooking

edamame and

PEA
DIP

| 127 CALS | 8G FAT | 8G CARBS | 6G PROTEIN |

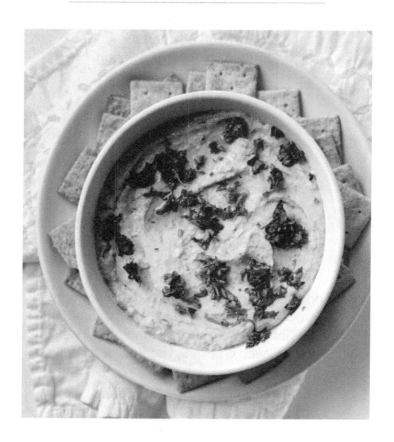

Edamame and Pea Dip

Recipe makes 6 servings

Macros per serving:
| 127 cals - 8g fat - 8g carbs - 6g protein |

Ingredients:
1 cup peas
1 cup edamame
1 cup <u>dairy free plain yogurt</u>
3 cloves garlic
2 tbsp lemon juice
¼ cup parsley
2 tbsp nutritional yeast
2 tbsp olive oil
1 tsp salt

Recipe:
If using frozen edamame; bring a small pot of water
to boil and add frozen edamame beans
Allow to cook 7-8 minutes or until softened
Drain and rinse with cold water
Add everything to a high speed blender or food
processor and blended until super smooth
The longer you blend the smoother it gets!
Enjoy with crackers, veggies, or bread!

<u>*Increase the portion*</u>

Enjoy on toast with and additional protein source
like smokey tempeh or smoked tofu

Use it as a sauce over potatoes for a delicious side dish

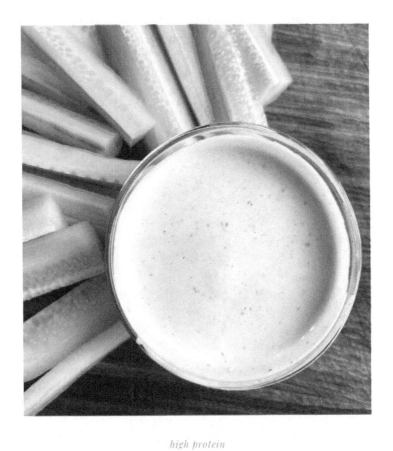

high protein

TAHINI
DIP

| 145 CALS | 11G FAT | 9G CARBS | 7G PROTEIN |

High Protein Tahini Dip

Recipe makes 4 servings

Macros per serving:
| 145 cals - 11g fat - 9g carbs - 7g protein |

Ingredients:
¼ cup tahini
½ cup water
3 tbsp nutritional yeast
2 tbsp hemp seeds
2 tbsp apple cider vinegar
1 tbsp maple syrup
1 tsp garlic powder
½ tsp salt

Recipe:
Add everything to a high speed blender and blend until smooth

Increase the portion

Make extra Buffalo Chickpea Balls and use this as the dip!

Use as a salad dressing to up the protein of your favorite greens

Final Thoughts

The protein-focused recipes in this cookbook, created to be easy to throw together, are loaded with flavor and colors. The goal is to make vegan food approachable and second nature to create. In a society where veganism isn't the norm (yet), it can be hard to figure out how to build a balanced plate that's still protein focused without the "usual" protein source.

This cookbook gives you a variety of ways to approach vegan protein that you may have never considered before, allowing you to sit and enjoy a meal feeling satisfied, energized, and never bloated.

The goal of the cookbook is to teach you some staple ideas so you can continue eating a healthy, mostly whole foods diet that is rich in protein so you can build the physique you want without sacrifice.

If you enjoyed this cookbook, follow me on Instagram @evannryan. You can enjoy free daily high protein recipes, tips, and tricks, and we can engage on a personal level so I can help you reach your healthy eating potential.

This High Protein Vegan Meal Prep Cookbook is Volume One of many more cookbooks. Make sure to join the mailing list through my Instagram (link in bio) to be notified of the next launch!

Happy meal prepping!

Made in the USA
Las Vegas, NV
10 November 2023

80538789R10059